The Top 20
Most Valuable
Herbs

The Top 20 Most Valuable Herbs

By Monica Sidoine,
S.N.H.S. Dip. Herbalism

DISCLAIMER

This book is to serve as an informational guide for use in the home. The remedies and procedures contained in this book are meant to supplement and are not intended to be a substitute for professional medical care. Please seek a qualified medical practitioner for all ailments. The author nor distributors takes no responsibility for customers choosing to treat themselves. Your use of this information is at your own risk.

ISBN - 13: 978-1534887961
ISBN - 10: 1534887962

Proof Read by Jasmine Ned Anunda

Printed By Create Space Publishing
United States of America

ACKNOWLEDGMENTS

I would like to thank all those who have contributed in one way or another to the completion of "THE TOP 20 MOST VALUABLE HERBS."

I thank God for giving me the vision, wisdom and good health to write this book. For all he has done and will continue to do in my life.

For the many prayer warriors who interceded on behalf of this project and also their moral support.

I thank my daughter Jasmine Ned Anunda for proof reading.

Thank you all.

Monica Sidoine.

PREFACE

Herbalism is the study and use of plants, mainly herbs and their medicinal uses.

Herbalism covers a great range of activity. Herbs are used in horticulture, cosmetics, medicine, cuisine, ornamentation and lots of other areas.

In days past when people lived more in tune with nature they were very aware of the importance of plants in their day to day lives. However with the changes over the years many persons have sought to the quick fix method. There are still many persons who prefer the natural way which is always the best.

The herbs presented in this book are the Top 20 most valuable herbs which you should have in your cupboard. You might not be able to have all of them but having a few would still be good. They would come in very handy when the need arises.

TABLE OF CONTENTS

GATHERING HERBS

The best time to gather herbs is on a bright day when there is no humidity. Allow the dew to clear off and the sun to warm up the weather.

- Take along a book with the photos of the plants that you need so that you will pick the correct plants. It is better to be on the safe side.

- Do not gather plants which are very close to the roadside due to the pollution from vehicles or industrial businesses.

- Do not gather plants close to farms due to the pesticides and herbicides which the farmers might be using in their produce.

- Inspect the plants first before picking them to make sure that they were not bitten by insects and that they are fit to be used.

- Do not gather too much from one particular place so as not to destroy the lot.

- Do not uproot the entire plant, only take the part that you need.

- When collecting plants it is better to put them separately in paper bags because they can sweat if they are in nylon bags.

- Flowers – Gather them when they are about to open.

- Leaves – Gather them before the flowers are in full bloom.

- Stems – Gather them after the appearance of the leaves but before the flowers grow.

- Bark – Gather them in the spring before flowering begins.

- Roots and Rhizomes – Gather them in autumn when the leaves have fallen.

DRYING HERBS

After you have taken the time to pick the plants, you now have to make sure that you do your best in getting them dried in the proper way so as not to lose them.

- Find a suitable location for drying the plants, clean and well aired with shade.

- Do not allow them to be in direct sunlight.

- Make sure that the plants are not moist to attract any form of bacteria.

- Spread them out in thin layers on white paper.

- Give them a little shake or turning twice during the day.

- The flowers can be tied in bunches and hung upside down.

- The fruits can be placed in a tray but will have to be turned constantly during the day so that they will not spoil and to get an even drying.

- If the weather is hot the drying can take up to eight days for flowers and up to six days for leaves. If it is cold it will take more time than that.

- Throughout the drying process they can be placed in the sun for a short time to prevent any fungus from developing.

STORING HERBS

After the herbs have been properly dried now is the time to store them properly so that they will not spoil or lose their medicinal properties.

- The herbs can be best stored in a brown paper bag or a glass bottle.

- Herbal oils will have to be stored in dark bottles.

- They should be labeled with the name and the date when they were packaged.

- Storage should be in a dry airy room.

- A shelf life of one year is good however if it is properly sealed with wax it can stay up to two years.

INFUSIONS

An infusion is an herbal tea.

It is used for parts that are easy to extract the medicinal qualities out of like leaves and flowers, example peppermint leaves or chamomile flowers and powdered bark.

An Infusion can be made with cold water, a sun tea or using boiling water.

A basic formula for making an Infusion is:-

Use 1 teaspoonful of dried herb or 2 teaspoons of fresh herb to the cup of water, or 1oz of herb to 1 liter of water.

Hot Infusion:
Pour the boiling water over the herbs, cover and let it steep for 15-30 minutes.

Cold Infusion:
Soak the herbs in cold water for 4 hours.

Sun Tea:
Pour water over the herbs and place it in the sun for 4 hours.

DECOCTIONS

A Decoction is also an herbal tea.

It is used for the harder parts of herbs such as the barks, roots, twigs, berries, fruit, nuts, hard seeds etc.

A basic formula for making a Decoction is:-

Add 1/2 to 1oz or 1 to 4 tablespoons of dried herb to 1 liter of cold water. Boil it for 30 minutes.

THE TOP TWENTY MOST VALUABLE HERBS

CAYENNE - Capsicum anuum

It stops heart attacks.
A tonic for the heart.
It is good for coughs, flus and colds.
It attracts blood to a body part.
It is good for indigestion.
Sluggish circulation.
It is good for varicose veins.
To enhance fertility.
It is good for aching legs.
It is useful for high or low blood pressure.
It is useful for arthritis, bronchitis and asthma.
It is good for painful joints and areas of swelling.
It stops bleeding when sprinkled on a bleeding cut.
It can be used as a fomentation for inflammation, wounds and rheumatism.

Method
- Steep ½ teaspoon in 2 cups of boiling water for 15 minutes. Drink 1 cup twice daily.

- Take 2 capsules three times daily.

  For as long as you feel it is necessary.
  Stop the treatment when you notice an improvement.

**N.B. Very excessive use can damage the kidneys.
It can cause dermatitis and raise blisters if it is applied to
the skin over a long period of time.**

CHARCOAL – Carbon

Charcoal is not an herb but it is very valuable and it is pure carbon.

It is good for diarrhea and hemorrhoids
It is good for colitis, cellulitis and hepatitis.
It adsorbs some poisons and it cleanses.
It is good for insect bites and wounds.
It is good for earaches and eye problems.
It is good for stomach aches and sore throat.
It is good for cancer, kidney infections and pain.
It is good for earaches and eye problems.
It is good for stomach aches and sore throat.
It is good for jaundice, allergic reactions, skin infections and rashes.
It is good for intestinal gas and it prevents intestinal infections.
It helps to reduce inflammation and elevated cholesterol; inflamed
fissures.
It is good for bad breath, abscess tooth, gum infection and sores in
the mouth.
It hastens the formation of the head in an abscess or a boil.
It deodorizes and disinfects.

Method
- Mix 1 teaspoon in 1 cup of water.
  Drink it and drink some more water after it.

- Take 8 tablets or 4 capsules daily.

   N.B. Drink it in the mid-morning or afternoon, not with your meals because the food will interfere with the effectiveness of it, it will increase the speed of digestion and the nutrients may be lost.
   Take it 12 hours after using prescription drugs.

- It can also be used as a poultice for bee stings, skin infections, wounds and kidney infections.

- It can be used as a fomentation for pain.

- It can be used as an enema for infections, ulcers and viral diseases.

- It can be used in the bath water for skin infections.

GARLIC - Allium sativum

Dissolves and Removes Tumors.
It detoxifies the body.
It is an expectorant.
It is good for diabetes.
It is good for cancer prevention.
Good for High Blood Pressure.
It is good for blood circulation.
Kills Candida Yeast Infection.
Stimulates the Lymphatic System.
It is good for coughs, colds and sore throats.

Dissolves Cholesterol in the bloodstream.
It helps with sinus congestion, bronchitis and asthma.
It regularizes the action of the gallbladder and the liver.
An antibiotic and helps to strengthen the immune system.
Used externally for ringworms and warts.

Method

- Take 1 tablespoon of garlic syrup three times daily.

- Take 5 capsules three times daily.

- Chew 3 raw cloves three times daily.

- It can be made into a syrup for coughs and colds.

- It can be used as a poultice.

   N.B. Persons who are on blood thinning drugs should not take it.

GOLDENSEAL - Hydrastis Canadensis

It helps to relieve morning sickness.
It is good for allergies.
It is good for prostate and liver problems.
It is good for alcoholism.
It is good for swollen hemorrhoids.
It strengthens the immune system.
It decreases uterine bleeding.
It is used for herpes and infections.

It is good for diabetes, eczema and chicken pox.
It is good for tonsillitis.
It is good for vaginal infections.
It is good for colds, bronchitis, asthma, flus, sore throat, and bad breath.

Method

- Steep 1oz of the powder in 1 liter of boiling water for 15 minutes.
  Take 1 teaspoon three times daily.

- Take 2 capsules three times daily.

- It can be used as a fomentation for skin infections.

- It can be used as a gargle for throat problems especially tonsillitis.

- It can be used as a douche for vaginal infections.

- It can be used as an enema to help reduce swollen hemorrhoids.

  N. B. Do not use it if you have high blood pressure or insomnia.
  Use it one week at a time.
  Don't use if you normally have miscarriages.
  Don't use in big quantities if you are hypoglycemic.

PEPPERMINT - Mentha piperita

It is good for gas and diarrhea.
Reduces Fevers.
It helps with insomnia.
Increases Circulation.
It is good for sinusitis.
Contains Antioxidants that help fight cancer and heart disease.
Strengthens heart muscle and calms the nerves.
The oil brings oxygen into the bloodstream.
It is good for menstrual cramps and muscle spasms.
It eases the spasm of irritable bowel syndrome.
It is good for morning sickness vomiting and nausea.
It eases the pain of congested varicose veins.
It helps with headaches and migraines.
Aids digestion and relieves indigestion.
Cleanses and strengthens the entire Body.

Method

- Steep 1oz to 1 pint of boiling water for 15 minutes. Drink 1 cup twice daily.

- Take 10 capsules three times daily.

- It can be added to the bath water for itchy skin infection.

- For a steam inhalation, 5 drops of the oils can be added to the water, which is good for treating sinusitis.

ECHINACEA - Echinacea angustifolia

It is an antibiotic.
A good blood and lymphatic cleanser.
It is an antiseptic agent and antimicrobial.
It helps with the recovery of the immune system.
Aids digestion and is a digestive tonic.
Venereal disease and viral infections. E.g. syphilis, vaginal infections, gonorrhea.
Inflammation of the mammary glands and skin diseases.
Bad breath, tonsillitis and insect bites.

Method

- Simmer 1oz of the root in 1 liter of water for 15 minutes. Drink 1 tablespoon six times daily.

- Take 2 capsules three times daily.

- It can be used as a fomentation for acne, swollen parts of the body and also open wounds.

- It can be used as a douche for vaginal infections.

  N.B. Pregnant persons, persons allergic to plants from the sunflower family or ragweed please use with caution. Persons with autoimmune disorders only take it for one week at a time.

CASCARA SAGRADA - Rhamnus purshiana

It helps with indigestion.

Good for intestinal gas.
It is good for jaundice.
It is a laxative for chronic constipation.
Liver and gallbladder problems.

Method

- Simmer 1oz of the bark in 1 liter of water for 15 minutes. Drink 1 cup daily.

- Take 3 capsules twice daily.

CATNIP - Nepata cataria

It reduces nervous tension.
Good for insomnia and fevers.
Gas and stomach cramps in children and infants.
It is good for diarrhea.
Stimulates the appetite.
Good for colds and bronchitis,
It is good for dizziness, morning sickness and headaches.
It is good for expelling worms.
It aids in relaxing the bowels.
It is good for mumps and painful swellings.
Small pox and urine retention.

Method

- Steep 1oz in 1 liter of boiling water for 15 minutes. Drink 1 cup daily.

- Take 5 capsules three times daily.

- As an enema to expel worms and relax the bowels.

- As a fomentation for mumps and painful swellings.

CORN SILK - Zea mays

Increases urine flow.
Helps with kidney and bladder problems.
Prostate disorders.
Relieve mucus from the urine.
Decreases bed-wetting if it is taken a few hours before bedtime.
Chronic cystitis, kidney stones.
Excess uric acid, urine retention.

Method
Steep 1oz in 1 liter of boiling water for 15 minutes.
Drink 3oz when the need arises.

HOPS - Humulus lupulus

Insomnia and restlessness.
Stimulates the appetite.
Weak nerves, anxiety, pain
It calms the mood.
It is a potent antispasmodic.
Sexually transmitted diseases.
It is a hangover remedy.
Coughs, fevers and chest ailments.

Relieves intestinal cramps and gas.
Cardiovascular disorders.
Jaundice, ulcers, toothaches.
Externally for boils, earaches.
It eases digestive inflammations and increases digestion.
When it is applied externally it has a local antiseptic effect.

Method
- Steep 1oz in 1 liter of boiling water for 15 minutes. Drink 1 cup three times daily.

- Take 5 capsules three times daily.

- Eat 6 flowers with 1 teaspoon of honey morning and night.

- It can be used as a fomentation for earaches, bruises, ulcers, boils, skin infections and inflammation.

- It can be used as a poultice with bran or wheat flour added to it for binding. To be used for drawing infections and abscesses.

- An herbal hop pillow can be made to be used for treating insomnia.

COMFREY - Symphytum officinale

Aids digestion.
Blood purifier.
Gallbladder inflammation.

Asthma, coughs and lung troubles.
Internal bleeding.
Regulates blood sugar levels.
Anemia, arthritis and bronchitis.
It eases joints that are aching.
It soothes muscles that are strained.
It encourages healing of ulcers on the legs.
It speeds up the knitting of bone.
Externally it heals fractures, sores, ulcers, rashes, sunburns, scabies, nosebleeds, bleeding and wounds.

Method

- Steep 1oz of the leaves in 1 liter of boiling water for 30 minutes.
  Drink 1 cup three times daily.

- Simmer 1oz of the root in 1 liter of water for 30 minutes.
  Drink ½ cup three times daily.

- Take 5 capsules three times daily.

- The leaves can be used as a poultice for burns, wounds, open sores, moist ulcers and also gangrene.

- It can be used as a fomentation for sunburns, skin infections, bedsores and insect bites.

- It can be used as a mouthwash for healing mouth ulcers and soothing gum diseases.

- It can be used as an ointment for bruises.

- It can be used as a hair rinse for sensitive scalp.

FLAXSEED - Linum usitatissimum

Gas,
It eases tiredness.
Stomach ulcers.
Hemorrhoids.
Eliminates gallstones.
All intestinal inflammations.
Asthma, bronchitis.
Lung and chest problems.
Constipation, diarrhea and it is a good laxative.
It is good for soothing a dry or rasping cough.
It eases spasm from irritable bowel syndrome.
It helps with the flushing of menopause.

Method
- Steep 1oz in 1 liter of boiling water for 15 minutes. Drink 1 cup daily.

- Simmer 1oz in 1 liter of water for 20 minutes. Drink ¼ cup three times daily.

- Drink 3 capsules daily.

- For constipation eat 2 tablespoons of the seeds. Drink lots of water after and then eat a few stewed prunes.

- As a poultice for burns, sores, tumors, inflammations and for drawing an infection to a head.

  N.B. Please avoid it if you are suffering with diverticulitis.

GINGER - Zingiberis officinalis

Scanty urine
Cleanses the colon.
Inflammation and arthritis.
Reduces spasms and cramps.
Reduces flatulent colic.
Contagious diseases.
Muscle aches, pain, gas and hot flashes.
Coughs, colds, sore throat, fever and sinus congestion.
Morning sickness, vomiting, motion sicknesses and nausea.
Stimulates the flow of saliva, digestion and circulation.

Method
- Steep 1oz in 1 liter of boiling water for 15 minutes. Drink 1oz at a time.

- Simmer 1oz of the root in 1 liter of water for 15 minutes. Drink ¼ cup three times daily.

- Take 2 capsules three times daily.

- It can be used as a fomentation for mumps.

SLIPPERY ELM - Ulmus fulva

A cleanser.
Gas and ulcers.
Ovarian cramps.
Bladder inflammation.
Constipation and diarrhea.

Colitis, cystitis, tonsillitis and bronchitis.
Lung congestion, flu, coughs and hoarseness.
Externally for sores, tumors, burns, hemorrhoids.

Method

- Steep 1oz in 1 pint of boiling water for 15 minutes.
  Drink 1 cup three times daily.

- Simmer 1oz of the inner bark in 1 liter of water for 20 minutes.
  Drink ½ cup three times daily.

- It can be used as a fomentation for burns, open sores, wounds, tumors and hemorrhoids.

- It can be used as a thin boiled cereal for the sick and elderly who are experiencing weak stomachs; also for children.

- It can also be used in a douche or enema.

WITCH HAZEL - Hamamelis virginiana

Diarrhea.
Hemorrhoids.
Varicose veins.
Uterine problems.
Stops excessive menstruation.
Stops bleeding from the uterus, lungs and other internal organs.
Externally for minor burns, insect bites, sore breasts and muscles; and bed sores.

Method

- Steep 1oz of leaves in 1 liter of boiling water for 15 minutes. Drink 1 cup whenever the need arises.

- Simmer 1oz of bark in 1 liter of water for 20 minutes. Drink 1 cup twice daily.

- It can be used as a vaginal douche.

- It can be used as a poultice for varicose veins, hemorrhoids and eye inflammation.

- It can be used as a fomentation for bedsores, eyes which are sore and inflamed; and skin infections.

- It can be used in a Sitz Bath three times a week for treating hemorrhoids.

- It can be used as a mouthwash for inflamed gums and sore throat by adding 3 drops of peppermint oil to the solution.

- A soaked squeezed cotton pad of the tea placed over the eyes will help to reduce puffiness and refresh the eyes.

LOBELIA - Lobelia inflate

Lock-jaw.
A sedative and an expectorant.
Indigestion.
Heart palpitation.

Allergies, chicken pox and arthritis.
Toothaches and teething.
Relaxant and stimulant.
Relieves Cramps and Spasms.
Balances glands for proper function.
Asthma, whooping cough, lung and respiratory conditions.
Superior remedy for fevers, headaches, pneumonia and jaundice.

Method
- Steep 1oz in 1 liter of boiling water for 15 minutes.
  Drink 1 tablespoon when the need arises.

- It can be used as a poultice for sprains, bruises, ringworm, muscle spasm, snake and insect bites, tumors and poison ivy.

- It can be used in the bath water or as a fomentation for skin diseases and muscle spasms.

- It can be used in a liniment for muscle spasms, sore muscles, pain and rheumatism.

- For earache you can put 2 drops of the tincture in the ear.

  N.B. Very large doses of it can be poisonous.

MYRRH - Commiphora mayrrha

It is an antiseptic, disinfectant, expectorant and a deodorizer.
A good stimulator for the immune system and gastric secretions.
Relieves asthma, sinusitis, sore throat, coughs.
Removes toxins from the stomach and the intestine.

Ulcers, sores, mouth sores, thrush, skin diseases, bed sores, boils.
Lung disease, chronic diarrhea, weakness
Hemorrhoids

Method
- Steep 1oz of the gum in 1 liter of boiling water for 15 minutes.
  Drink ½ cup three times daily.

- Take 2 capsules three times daily.

- The tincture can be used for treating oral infections and gum boils.

- Use it as a wash for skin diseases and wounds.

   N.B. Do not use large amounts for a long period.

SKULLCAP - Scutellaria lateriflora

Insanity.
Hyperactivity.
It strengthens the heart.
It is an effective relaxant.
It is an antispasmodic herb.
It helps with indigestion.
It is very good for nerve problems.
It reduces ovarian or uterine pains.
It helps to promote menstruation.
It helps with symptoms due to drug and alcoholic withdrawal.

Assists with insomnia, fatigue, anxiety, stress, muscle cramps, pain, headaches, epilepsy, and coughs.

Method
- Steep 1oz of the tops in 1 liter of boiling water for 20 minutes.
  Drink 1 cup four times daily.

- Take 3 capsules twice daily.

- It can also be used in a Sitz Bath three times a week for treating anxiety.

  N.B. It should not be used too regularly. Since there is a suspected risk of it causing liver impairment.

VERVAIN - Verbena officinalis

Lung ailments.
Induce sweating.
Increase mother's milk.
Convulsions.
Good for eliminating intestinal worms.
Rheumatism and sciatica,
Bowel pains and intestinal cramps.
Headaches, measles.
It is good for nervous problems, mild depression and insomnia.
Reduce fevers, colds, coughs, throat and chest congestions, pneumonia, asthma, and upper respiratory inflammations.

Method

- Steep 1oz of the tops in 1 liter of boiling water for 15 minutes.
  Drink ½ cup four times daily.

- It can be used as a fomentation on wounds, sores and for toothaches.

- It can be used as a poultice with wheat flour added to it for binding and placed on the swollen part of the spleen.

  N.B. Do not use it if you are pregnant.
  It is poisonous if taken in large doses.

RED CLOVER - Trifolium pretense

Dissolves and removes tumors.
Powerful remedy for Cancer growth.
Excellent blood and lymphatic cleanser.
Thins the Blood.
Improves Circulation.
Stops spasms.
Good for whooping cough.
Induces expectoration
An appetite suppressor.
Strengthens the immune system.
Good for lack of vitality and nervous energy.
Is a tonic for the nerves and a sedative for nervous exhaustion.
Bronchitis, kidney problems, inflamed lungs, liver disease.
Rheumatism, HIV, AIDS, psoriasis, bacterial infections

Method

- Steep 1oz of the flowering tops in 1 liter of boiling water for 30 minutes.
  Drink 1 cup four times daily.

- It can be used as a poultice or a fomentation on areas with cancerous growths.

INDEX OF HERBS

INDEX OF HERBS

Other Book Titles by the Same Author

Can be viewed at this link:
http://www.amazon.com/author/monicasidoine

Healing Poultices

Home Remedies For Cancer

Home Remedies For Losing Weight

Home Remedies For Blood Pressure and Diabetes

Home Remedies For Headaches and Insomnia

Home Remedies For Stress, Depression and Anxiety

Home Remedies For Constipation and Diarrhea

Home Remedies For Asthma and Bronchitis

Home Remedies For Dehydration and Vomiting

Home Remedies For Pneumonia and Tuberculosis

Home Remedies For Sinusitis and Tonsillitis

Home Remedies For Heart Attack and Strokes

Home Remedies For Colds, Fever and Sore Throat

NOTES

NOTES

NOTES